Herbalism:

A Complete Reference Guide to Frequently used Magickal Herbs, and Spices

By: Kristina Benson

Herbalism: A Complete Reference Guide to Frequently used Magickal Herbs, and Spices

ISBN 13: 978-1-60332-034-4

Table of Contents

Herbalism

INTRODUCTION

It was only in the last century that ailing, injured, or sick people would turn to various herbs and foodstuffs for help before turning to a doctor or pharmacy. Of course, doctors and pharmacies have wonderful drugs and methods to give in order to heal us. But the ability to heal ourselves from minor--or occasionally even major—ailments still is very much within our own kitchen or grocery store.

For some reason, over the course of the last century, the knowledge of herbal medicine and home remedies has been lost and obfuscated. We have come to regard pharmaceutical companies as the sole purveyors of well-being. Though it is very much in their interest for us to believe as such, the reality is that we are perfectly capable of healing ourselves much of the time without their help.

In this book, I have made an effort to include herbs and foodstuffs that are easy to find, and that many households stock on a regular basis. I have included some recipes, as well as a glossary. Of course, this book should not substitute for professional medical care. IT can, however, act as a useful supplement.

The first, and largest section, covers each food or herb, what it can be used for, and what its main properties are.

The next is a glossary, followed by a cautionary section for pregnant women. This is followed by some of my favorite recipes and home remedies.

I hope you enjoy and prosper from this book!

GATHERING HERBS

If you are fortunate enough to live in an area that has wild herbs growing for the picking, it will be a treat to pick them! What follows is a guide to gathering herbs, and then storing and drying them.

Remember, IF YOU DID NOT PLANT THE HERB YOURSELF, DO NOT USE IT FOR CONSUMPTION UNLESS YOU ARE 100% SURE YOU KNOW WHAT IT IS. This may seem obvious enough that it shouldn't need to be stated here, however, remember that a tiny variance in certain herbs may only be noticeable after careful comparison, or even expert evaluation. If you have even a tiny little doubt, don't pick it for consumption.

The Best Time for Gathering Plants

Whether or not you planted them yourself, it is important to gather herbs, bark, and plants at the correct time. First, know which part of the plant you will be using—the bark, the flowers, the leaves, or the roots.

  * barks should be gathered in the spring,
  * leaves should be collected before the plant flowers,

* flowers are best when picked on the first day of opening, and

* roots are best in the autumn, although you may in some cases harvest the roots before the plant has developed or reached maturity. Also, when collecting a root, make sure you get the entire root. A garden trowel or spade is essential when collecting roots.

A day without rain which has been sunny since sunrise is your best bet. If it's too hot, the oils can be dried out. So it is best to gather the leaves before the hottest part of the day. Try to pick leaves that are consistent in shape and color. If a leaf has been eaten partially by an insect, is discolored, or withered, don't use it. If you are harvesting the whole plant, as opposed to just the leaves, you will most likely have perfectly consistent, well-shaped leaves with a minimal amount of discoloration or stains.

When gathering leaves and flowers, don't kill off the plant that has been hosting it. Use garden scissors to remove the leaves or parts that you need. If you merely rip the leaf or stem out of the plant, you can leave the plant vulnerable to infection, or it can die.

When gathering the herbs in the wild be sure that you gather them in an area that is not sprayed with pesticides, and preferably far away from a road. Of course, plants growing near any sort of industry are probably not terribly desirable and are best left alone.

Protect the area from over-harvesting by leaving at least 3/4 of the plants intact for reproduction. If you gather an entire plant, make an effort to replant a seed, even if you are taking the plant from the wild.

DRYING HERBS

After you have gathered the herbs, it is in important that you prepare them to be dried as soon as possible. Gently wash the plants and pat them dry with a towel.

Herbs leaves, stems, and flowers should be dried by spreading them in single layers on a flat drying surface. Wire cooling racks can come in handy for this but if you don't have a wire cooling rack, a cookie sheet or a surface where the plants won't be disturbed is fine.

The drying can be done in the sunlight or the shade. The shade takes longer but it does seem to preserve more of the herb's potency. You can also dry herbs in paper bags so long as you barely have any plants in there. Otherwise they could just rot. It is also important to make sure that the bag has ventilation. Check the paper bags in about a week and if the herbs are not getting papery to the touch, spread them on a flat surface in a dry, dark area. Then they will dry before they can be compromised by molds resulting from moisture.

The amount of time that they need to dry will vary according to the plant and the conditions. If it is particularly hot and dry, the herbs may dry too quickly, especially if they are in the direct sunlight. If it is humid or overcast or foggy, you may have to put them in an oven on a very low temperature. Otherwise, the plants will become damp and vulnerable to molds and fungi.

Roots can be incredibly stubborn and it takes some effort to make sure that they dry properly. They may need to be gently scrubbed and rinsed of the soil, and the small rootlets removed. Large, thick roots can be sliced to get them to dry quicker.

When they have been washed and trimmed, they should be gathered and tied with a string. Turn and inspect them every day, and keep in mind that they will shrink considerably as they dry.

When the herb is dried (whether root, leaves stem or flower) they should be placed into a dry container, and handled carefully lest they break. They should ideally be stored in an amber glass container, as oils can permanently permeate a wooden box or ceramic vase. If you must use ceramic, make sure it is dark in color, an dglazed. Make sure you label the herb, and store it away from sunlight.

HERBS AND FOOD STUFFS

The following section is a guide to the most frequently used herbs and food stuffs.

ALOE VERA

Aloe vera syn. A. barbadensis (Liliaceae)

HISTORY and USES:

Though native to Africa, *aloe vera* can easily be cultivated elsewhere. The clear gel found inside the plant's leaf and alongside the leaf blade contains *aloin*, and can be used for medicinal and cosmetic purposes. The clear gel is an excellent soother and healer of wounds and burns, accelerating rate of healing and reducing the risk of infection. The brownish part containing *aloin* also is a strong laxative, and can be used effectively for short-term constipation. Aloe is present in many cosmetics' formulae because its emollient and scar preventing properties.

MAIN PROPERTIES:

Emollient, laxative, vulnerary

ANISE

Pimpinella anisum (Umbelliferae)

HISTORY and USES:

Anise has been cultivated in Egypt and was used for medicinal purposes by the Greeks, Romans and Arabs, who named the plant *anysun*. Since antiquity it has been used in Greece and in the cradle of civilization as a cooking spice, a diuretic, an agent used to treat digestive problems, and a analgesic for toothaches. Anise seeds are still used to reduce flatulence and colic, and to settle the digestion, and can be taken safely by both adults and children. Anise can also act as an expectorant and an antispasmodic that is helpful in soothing menstrual pain, asthma, whooping cough and bronchitis. Anise seeds also have mild hormonal action that is useful in increasing breast-milk production for lactating mothers. It has also been used for easing the pain of childbirth, and for treating impotence and encouraging sexual desire in both sexes. Anise essential oil is also very useful externally to treat lice and scabies.

MAIN PROPERTIES:

Reduces colic and flatulence, promotes digestion, antispasmodic

APPLE

Malus domestica

HISTORY and USES:

Apples are one of the most widely cultivated and consumed fruits. Research suggests that the consumption of apples may reduce the risk of colon cancer, prostate cancer and lung cancer. Apples also contain a naturally occurring antioxidant that has shown some promise in protecting cells from the effects of stress

Apple consumption can help remove food stuck between the teeth, but the acid contained in the fruit is also capable of eroding tooth enamel over time, so eating an apple should not be a substitute for tooth brushing. Raw, overripe, or baked apple can be made into a poultice to treat a sprain, or put over the eyes to relieve eyestrain. Apple water can also reduce a fever.

MAIN PROPERTIES:

Febrifuge, astringent, antioxidant source

APPLE CIDER VINEGAR

HISTORY and USES:

Apple cider vinegar, available at most grocery stores, is an excellent supplement to any natural medicine cabinet. It can reduce inflammation, bruising and swelling. Apple cider vinegar has also been said to be instrumental cancer prevention, and is affective in the alleviation of joint pain, and weight loss. Claims of its benefits go back at least to Hippocrates. Many believe that vinegar is also a cure to mild to moderate sunburn. Cider vinegar is also claimed to be a solution to dandruff, and a natural remedy for yeast infections, when diluted with water and used as a douche.

MAIN PROPERTIES:

Astringent, anti-inflammatory.

APRICOT/APRICOT SEED

Prunus armeniaca

HISTORY and USES:

The apricot fruit comes from a tree that is thought to have originated in China, and was brought to Europe by the Moors when they invaded and took over Spain.

Laetrile, which has long been considered a treatment for cancer, is extracted from apricot seeds. As early as the year 502, apricot seeds were used to treat tumors and ulcers. The American Medical Association, however, does not substantiate the effectiveness of laetrile.

Apricots have also been used as an aphrodisiac, and to stimulate uterine contractions.

MAIN PROPERTIES:

Emmenagogue, aphrodisiac

ARNICA

Arnica

HISTORY and USES:

Arnica is a genus that contains about thirty plants, and is in the sunflower family. There are a few species native to Eurasia, but most occur in North America..

In herbal medicine, Arnica usually refers to Arnica Montana, used for relief of bruises, stiffness, and muscle soreness. It is available in natural/health food stores, in gel or tablet form, to be taken internally or to be applied to the affected area.

MAIN PROPERTIES:

anti-inflammatory, analgesic, relaxant.

ARROWROOT

Maranta arundinacea (Marantaceae)

HISTORY and USES:

Arrowroot is native to South America and the Caribbean. The indigenous peoples in these areas have long used its root as a poultice for sores, and as an infusion to treat urinary tract infections. It can also be used as a soothing agent on inflamed mucous membrane tissue, a nutrient in convalescence, and for easing digestion. It helps to relieve acidity, indigestion and colic, and can act as a gentle laxative. It may be applied as an ointment, demulcent, or poultice mixed with some other antiseptic herbs such as comfrey.

MAIN PROPERTIES:

Anti-inflammatory, digestive, antiseptic.

ANGELICA

Angelica arcangelica (Umbelliferae)

HISTORY and USES:

Angelica has been used in herbal medicine since the fifteenth century, and continues to be a very helpful herb to this day. Angelica can reduce spasms resulting from asthma and bronchitis. It has also been shown to ease rheumatic inflammation, to regulate menstrual flow, and to stimulate the appetite. The stems can also be very useful for culinary purposes.

MAIN PROPERTIES:

Antispasmodic, promotes menstrual flow, appetite stimulant.

ARNICA

Arnica montana (Compositae)

HISTORY and USES:

Arnica has been used extensively in European folk medicine. Goethe, the famous poet and philosopher, used arnica to ease symptoms of angina. Arnica extracts, ointments and compresses can be used to reduce inflammation and pain resulting from bruises, sprains, dislocations, and swelling, and can also ease general tendon and muscle aches. Arnica improves circulation and accelerates healing. It is an anti-inflammatory and can be helpful to stop internal bleeding. Extreme caution should be used in ingesting arnica as it can be toxic.

MAIN PROPERTIES:

Anti-inflammatory, germicide, muscular soreness, pain reliever

ARTEMISIA, WORMWOOD

Artemisia absinthium (Compositae)

HISTORY and USES:

The name of this plant comes from the Roman word for "bitter". As such, this herb has been used to flavor drinks. Wormwood has a tonic effect on the stomach and the gallbladder and is helpful in treating mild digestive problems. It can be used to get rid of roundworms and threadworms, and can help alleviate the symptoms of anemia. It is also a muscle relaxant used to treat rheumatism and muscle spasms. The leaves of wormwood have antiseptic properties. Wormwood can also have a narcotic effect, and as such, caution should be used in ingesting this herb.

MAIN PROPERTIES:

To add flavor, carminative, sedative, antiseptic, vermifuge

ASTRALAGUS

Astralgus alpinus, astralagus glycyphyllos

HISTORY and USES:

This is a tonic herb originally used in Chinese medicine. It is believed to promote lactation in nursing mothers, and recent studies show that it may strengthen the human immune system.

The natural gum tragacanth, which is used today in pharmaceuticals and textiles, is from Astragalus tragacanthus. The Chinese used the many varieties of Astralagus to promote the discharge of pus and speed healing, even out spikes in blood sugar associated with diabetes, and as a diuretic. In western herbal medicine, Astragalus is primarily considered a tonic for enhancing metabolism and digestion. It is usually consumed as a tea made from the roots of the plant.

MAIN PROPERTIES:

Diuretic, boost metabolism, strengthen immune system, and promote wound healing.

BASIL, HOLY BASIL

Ocimum sanctum (Labiatae)

HISTORY and USES:

Holy basil, like the basil commonly used in cooking, comes from India. The Egyptians used basil in holy settings, burning a mixture of basil and myrrh to appease their gods. Sweet Basil—the basil we use for culinary purposes to this day--was later introduced in Europe as a seasoning. Though obviously useful in the kitchen, the herb has widespread medicinal properties. Most notable is its ability to even out spikes in blood sugar levels. It also prevents peptic ulcers and other stress related conditions like hypertension, colitis and asthma. Basil is also used to treat a cold, and reduce fevers, congestion and joint pain. Basil leaves can act as both an antiseptic and a fungicide, and as such, basil leaves can bring relief to itching skin, the sites of insect bites, and rashes.

MAIN PROPERTIES:

Lowers blood sugar levels, antispasmodic, analgesic, lowers blood pressure, febrifuge, fungicidal, anti-inflammatory.

BEET

beta vulgaris

HISTORY and USES:

Though the root is used for cooking in the west, it is possible to use the tops of the beet as salad greens. The root is extremely versatile, and can be peeled, steamed or baked, and then eaten warm with butter; or peeled, shredded raw, and then eaten as a salad. The Romans used beet root as a treatment for fevers and constipation, to bind wounds, and as an aphrodisiac.

MAIN PROPERTIES:

Aphrodisiac, laxative, vulnerary

BELLADONA/ DEADLY NIGHTSHADE

Atropa belladonna (Solanaceae)

HISTORY and USES:

Deadly nightshade is native to Europe, western Asia and northern Africa. *Herba bella dona*, or "herb of the beautiful lady" can accelerate the heart rate and cause death if used improperly, but can act as an important and beneficial healing agent when used correctly. Belladonna contains *atropine,* a chemical used in modern, western ophthalmology to dilate the pupils for eye examinations, and is also used as an anesthetic. In herbal or holistic medicine, deadly nightshade is mainly used to relieve intestinal colic, to treat peptic ulcers and to relax distended digestive organs.

MAIN PROPERTIES:

Anesthetic, antispasmodic, narcotic, reduces sweating, sedative.

BENZOIN GUM

Styrax benzoin (Styraceae)

HISTORY and USES:

Benzoin is a tree native to the southeastern part of Asia. In the center of its trunk is a gum well. The gum has strong astringent and antiseptic properties. For this reason it can be used externally to fight tissue inflammation and to disinfect. When ingested internally, benzoin gum can soothe pain, stimulate coughing, and alleviate urinary tract infections. It also is widely used in modern day cosmetics as an antioxidant in oils, as a fixative in perfumes, and as an additive to soaps. If the gum is boiled and the steam inhaled, the fumes calms inflammation in sore throats, loosens phlegm in head and chest colds, and treats asthma and bronchitis.

MAIN PROPERTIES:

Antiseptic, astringent, anti-inflammatory.

BERGAMOT

Citrus bergamia syn. C. aurantium var. bergamia
(Rutaceae)

HISTORY and USES:

The bergamot (*Citrus bergamia*) is a small pear-shaped citrus fruit indigenous to and grown mainly in Calabria Italy. Bergamot oil, expressed from the peel, can strengthen the immune system and help in avoiding infectious diseases. It is used in modern day cosmetics, and is useful in preventing oily skin, acne, psoriasis and acne. The oil is also sometimes added to sun-tanning oils. Bergamot essential oil can also be used to relieve tension, relax muscle spasms and improve digestion.

MAIN PROPERTIES:

Disinfectant, muscle relaxant.

BETONY

Stachys

HISTORY and USES:

There are about three hundred species that belong in the genus Stachys. They are native to Europe, and can be found growing in grasslands and woodland edges. Used as a medicine for centuries, betony is somewhat of a panacea. The whole plant is medicinal as alterative, antibacterial, antipyretic, antiseptic, antispasmodic, astringent, carminative, diuretic, febrifuge, hypotensive, stomachic, styptic, tonic, vermifuge and vulnerary. A cold water, weak infusion of the plant can act as amedicinal eye wash for sties and pinkeye. It is taken internally as a medicinal tea to treat fevers, diarrhea, sore mouth and throat, internal bleeding, and weaknesses of the liver and heart.

MAIN PROPERTIES:

alterative, antibacterial, antipyretic, antiseptic, antispasmodic, astringent, carminative, diuretic, febrifuge, hypotensive, stomachic, styptic, tonic, vermifuge and vulnerary.

BITTER ORANGE

Citrus aurantium (Rutaceae)

HISTORY and USES:

The bitter orange, native to tropical Asia, has been used as a source of food and medicine for thousands of years. Its oil has anti-inflammatory, antibacterial and antifungal properties. Bitter orange juice is rich in vitamin C, which can help strengthen the immune system and reduce the duration of a cold. As an infusion, it helps to relieve fever, and soothe headaches. *Neroli* oil can be expressed from its flowers, and the oil known as *petitgrain* from its leaves and young stalks. Both oils are used often in perfumery and in scented cosmetics. Orange flower water is a by-product of distillation and is to flavor breads and desserts, as well as being used to reduce heart rate and palpitations, to encourage sleep and calm the digestive tract.

MAIN PROPERTIES:

Source of vitamin C, anti-inflammatory, antifungal, antibacterial, carminative, febrifuge

BLACK COHOSH

Cimicifuga racemosa

HISTORY and USES:

Black cohosh has been used as a remedy for the symptoms of PMS and menopause. Some, however, feel that its benefits are largely due to a placebo effect. Recent research, however, suggests that it works by binding to serotonin receptors, rather than by mimicking the effects of estrogen, as had previously been thought. Native Americans used black cohosh to treat gynecological disorders, sore throats, kidney problems, and depression.

Black cohosh has been used also to induce abortion or miscarriage, and as such, should never be taken by lactating or pregnant women. It encourages blood flow to the pelvic region, and can, ergo, be helpful in cases of late menstruation.

MAIN PROPERTIES:

As a treatment for PMS, menopause, depression, late menstruation.

BOLDO

Peumus boldus (Umbelliferae)

HISTORY and USES

Boldo is a tree native to the Chilean Andes. It can act to stimulate the secretion and flow of saliva and gastric juices. *Boldine*, one of its ingredients, can eliminate the flow of bile, and has a protective effect on hepatic cells. Boldo stimulates liver activity and bile flow and is chiefly useful as a palliative for gallstones and liver or gallbladder pain. It is generally taken for a few weeks at a time, either as a tincture or infusion. Boldo also has antiseptic properties and can help in combating cystitis.

MAIN PROPERTIES:

Bile and liver activity stimulant, digestive

CABBAGE

HISTORY AND USES

Cabbages are flowering plants of the family Brassicaceae, and is related to the wild mustard plant. In European folk medicine, cabbage leaves are used to treat acute inflammation. One leaf can be dipped in water and placed on a wound in order to alleviate discomfort. It should be replaced after it gets warm from the wound. It also can help infected wounds and draw out pus in the same manner. One of the chemicals in cabbage can also treat respiratory papillomavirus.

MAIN PROPERTIES

Anti-inflammatory, vulnerary

CALENDULA, MARIGOLD

Calendula officinallis (Compositae)

HISTORY and USES:

Marigold is excellent for treating local skin problems. Infusions or decoctions of Calendula petals can act to decrease the inflammation resulting from sprains, stings, and varicose veins. It can also soothe burns, sunburns, rashes and general skin irritations. Decoctions, poultices, and infusions of marigold are excellent for treating inflamed and bruised skin, and have antiseptic and healing properties that can prevent the spread of infection and accelerate healing. Marigold is also a cleansing and detoxifying herb, and the infusion and tincture can treat infection. Taken internally, it can promote the draining of swollen lymph glands and relieve the symptoms of tonsillitis.

MAIN PROPERTIES:

Anti-inflammatory, astringent, vulnerary, antiseptic, detoxifier.

CAMPHOR

Cinnamomum camphora syn. Laurus camphora
(Lauraceae)

HISTORY and USES:

Camphor trees are native to China and Japan, and from the wood of these trees somce camphor oil. Marco Polo was the first westerner to note that the Chinese used camphor oil as a medicine, a scent in perfumery, and as embalming fluid. Camphor has very strong antiseptic, stimulant and antispasmodic properties and is applied externally to relieve arthritic and rheumatic pains, neuralgia and back pain. Generally, the camphor is made into a liniment. It may alleviate skin problems such as cold sores and chilblains, and used as an effective chest rub for bronchitis and other chest infections. To this day, Campho Phenique and Vicks, staples of the cold and flu section of any American drug store, use camphor essential oil as an active ingredient.

MAIN PROPERTIES:

Antiseptic, antispasmodic, analgesic, expectorant.

CANNABIS

Cannabis Sativa

HISTORY and USES:

There are many subspecies of this plant, and it should be noted that some are illegally to consume or cultivate in the United States. The flowers (and to a much lesser extent the leaves, stems, and seeds) contain psychoactive and physiologically active chemical compounds that have traditionally been consumed for recreational, medicinal, and religious purposes. The flowers, seeds, and stems can be ingested, smoked, vaporized, or made into ointments or teas. Smoking the flowers of the plant can stimulate the appetite and calm nausea. The hemp oil can soothe irritated or dry skin.

MAIN PROPERTIES:

Appetite stimulant, anti-nausea.

CARAWAY

Carum carvi

HISTORY and USES:

Caraway is native to Europe and Western Asia, and is commonly known in the West for its culinary uses. The plant has many medicinal properties, however. An herbal infusion made from the seeds is good for colic, loss of appetite, digestive disorders and to get rid of worms.

MAIN PROPERTIES:

Appetite stimulant, carminative, febrifuge

CARDAMOM

Elettaria cardamomum (Zingiberaceae)

HISTORY and USES:

Cardamom is useful as a culinary spice, a scent in perfumery, and as medicine and was used in ancient Egypt to make perfumes. Cardamom can act as a palliative for many digestive problems, and can help settle indigestion, dyspepsia, gastralgia, colon spasms and flatulence. It has an aromatic and distinctive taste and combines well with other herbs, particularly those with a pungent or bitter taste.

MAIN PROPERTIES:

Eases stomach pain, carminative, aromatic, antispasmodic.

CARDUS, MILK THISTLE, MARY THISTLE

Carduus marianus syn. Silybum marianum (Compositae)

HISTORY and USES:

Milk thistle is native to the Mediterranean and has been used for hundreds of years to help liver problems, including liver damage caused by excessive alcohol consumption. It is useful also for treating hepatitis, and for treating ailments of the bladder. Milk thistle has also been used to encourage the production of breast milk in lactating mothers, and can have some success as an antidepressants.

MAIN PROPERTIES:

Digestive, liver tonic, stimulates secretion of bile, increases breast-milk production, antidepressant.

CAYENNE PEPPER

Capsicum Solanaceae

HISTORY and USES:

Cayenne, consumed in powdered form, or as raw fruit, has been used as medicine for centuries. It is the most effective blood stimulant ever studied. In addition, it has endorphin-stimulating properties. It can treat stomachaches, cramping pains, and gas. If rubbed on the skin, it can act as an irritant, which, oddly enough, can be beneficial if rubbed on an area of the skin that has already been irritated. It can also be gargled as a wash to improve a sore throat. Some studies suggest that it can act as an appetite suppressant, and can help even out spikes in blood sugar. Cayenne peppers are also high in Vitamin C, Vitamin B, potassium, and iron.

MAIN PROPERTIES:

Expectorant, stimulant, appetite suppressant, blood thinner, irritant, anti-parasitic.

CELERY

Apium graveolens (Umbelliferae)

HISTORY and USES:

Although celery is now very common in culinary pursuits, it also has many fine healing properties. It's mainly used in the treatment of rheumatism, arthritis and gout. The seeds are also used as a urinary antiseptic. It is a very good cleansing herb, and a powerful diuretic, and can help in expelling waste and toxins. The seeds also have a reputation as a carminative with a mild tranquilizing effect. The stems are less significant medicinally, but are certainly useful in the kitchen.

MAIN PROPERTIES:

Anti-rheumatic, antispasmodic, diuretic, urinary antiseptic.

CHAMOMILE, GERMAN CHAMOMILE

Chamomilla recutita syn. Matricaria recutita
(Compositae)

HISTORY and USES:

The chamomile flower grows wild in Europe and west Asia, and similar species are found growing wild in North America and Africa. Its flowers help to ease indigestion, nervousness, depressions and headaches, and can help sufferers of peptic ulcers, colitis, spastic colon and nervous indigestion. Drinking a cup of hot chamomile tea at night can help restless sleepers or sufferers of insomnia, and chamomile essential oil, when used in a diffuser, can also inspire calm and sleepiness. Chamomile's essential oil has anti-inflammatory, anti-spasmodic and anti-microbial properties. It is an excellent herb for many digestive disorders and for nervous tension and irritability. Externally, it can be made into a poultice or salve and used for sore skin, rashes, sunburn, and eczema. Roman chamomile (Chamaemelum nobile) is a close relation, used in a similar way.

MAIN PROPERTIES:

Anti-inflammatory, antispasmodic, relaxant, carminative,

bitter, nerve tonic

CHICORY

Cicorium intybus (Compositae)

HISTORY and USES:

Chicory is native to Europe and has been used for medicine since the medieval times. As a tea or extract, chicory root is a digestive tonic that also increases bile flow and decreases inflammation in the digestive organs. The root can be roasted, and prepared in a manner that is very similar to coffee. The root can also aid in digestion, and clean out the urinary tract, preventing urinary tract infections. Chicory is also taken for rheumatic conditions and gout, and can be used a mild laxative. An infusion of the leaves and flowers also aids the digestion.

MAIN PROPERTIES:

Digestive, liver tonic, anti-rheumatic, mild laxative.

CINNAMON

Cinnamomum verum syn. C. zeylanicum (Lauraceae)

HISTORY and USES:

Cinnamon is native to Sri Lanka, and grows best in tropical forest climates. Cinnamon has long been used in India and Egypt for medicinal purposes. To this day, it is, of course, a common spice in cooking, and is used in perfumery. The infusion or powder is excellent to help alleviate stomach pains and cramps. There is also some evidence that cinnamon can help smooth out spikes in blood sugar. Cinnamon is also useful as a household insecticide and to keep away ants—if sprinkled on a trail of ants, the ants will die, and will be less likely to return. Traditionally, the herb was taken for colds, flu and digestive problems.

MAIN PROPERTIES:

Warming stimulant, carminative, antispasmodic, antiseptic, anti-viral, blood sugar regulator.

CLOVE

Eugenia caryophyllata syn. Syzgium aromaticum
(Myrtaceae)

HISTORY and USES:

Clove trees are native to India, and have long been used there for culinary and medicinal purposes. The dried flower buds, or the cloves, have a distinctive taste and a pleasant, though occasionally pungent, aroma. The buds, leaves and stems are used for the extractions of clove essential oil. The oil contains *eugenol*, which is a strong anesthetic and antiseptic substance. Cloves are also well known for their antispasmodic and simulative properties. Hot brandy with cloves and lemon juice can soothe sufferers of head and chest colds. The benefits of cloves do not, however, extend to consuming them as smoke. When smoked in pipes or as cigarettes, cloves actually cause more harm to the lung tissue than does tobacco.

MAIN PROPERTIES:

Antiseptic, mind and body stimulant, analgesic, antibacterial, carminative.

COMFREY

Symphytum officinale (Boraginaceae)

HISTORY and USES:

Comfrey's name derives from the Latin *con firma,* i.e. "with strength", as it was once believed to have the ability to heal broken bones. Though comfrey cannot, indeed, knit broken bones, the leaves and roots contain *allantoin,* an agent that accelerates the healing of wounds by acting to hasten cell multiplication. It can also be used in a poultice or salve to heal rashes, wounds, inflammation and skin problems. Internally, comfrey can soothe ulcers and colitis. It is also used for a variety of respiratory problems.

MAIN PROPERTIES:

Carminative, anti-inflammatory, vulnerary

COPTIS/GOLDENTHREAD

Coptis

HISTORY and USES:

These flowering plants are native to parts of Asia and North America, and have been a valuable part of Chinese herbalism for centuries. It is most often used as a bitter tonic for dyspepsia. It is also known to help insomnia in Chinese Medicine. If the flowers are made into a paste, balm, powder, or infusion, it is said to improve digestion, stimulate appetite, and relieve inflammation of the stomach. It is also said to be helpful in treating alcoholism.

MAIN PROPERTIES

Digestion, appetite stimulator, anti-inflammatory

CORIANDER

Coriandrum sativum (Umbelliferae)

HISTORY and USES:

Coriander has been used for medicinal purposes for over a thousand years, and is originally native to the Mediterranean and Caucasian regions. It can aid in digestion, reduce flatulence and stimulate the appetite. It can prevent spasms of the digestive organs, and prevent digestive problems caused by nervous disorders. Chewing coriander can also act as a natural breath freshener, even after consuming pungent foods like onions and garlic. Coriander can be applied externally as a lotion or balm to ease rheumatic pain. Coriander essential oil is still used in the manufacturing of perfumes, cosmetics, mouth washes, and toothpastes.

MAIN PROPERTIES:

Digestive, antispasmodic, anti-rheumatic, breath freshener.

CRANBERRY

Vaccinium erythrocarpum

HISTORY and USES:

Cranberries are a source of antioxidants and other phytochemicals that have been shown to offer tremendous benefit to the cardiovascular system and immune system. There is some evidence that these chemicals can also help fight and prevent cancer.

Drinking cranberry juice can prevent bacteria from flourishing in the urinary tract and bladder, and as such, can treat UTIs.

Cranberry juice, if consumed in an unsweetened form, has a chemical that can prevent and even reverse the formation of agents that cause tooth decay. Other chemicals in cranberries can help prevent kidney stones.

MAIN PROPERTIES

Antibacterial, anti-plaque

CUMIN

Nigella sativa

HISTORY and USES:

Cumin seeds have a bitter flavor and smell a bit like strawberries. It is a common household herb for cooking and flavoring liquor. Ibn Sina, known to westerners as Avicenna, refers to black cumin as a seed that stimulates the body's energy and helps recovery from fatigue and dispiritedness. He also describes it as having a positive effect on treating digestive disorders, gynecological diseases and respiratory ailments.

The seeds have been used in the Middle East and Southeast Asian countries to treat Asthma, Bronchitis, Rheumatism and related inflammatory diseases, to increase lactation, in nursing mothers, to promote digestion, and to fight parasitic infections. Its oil has been used to treat skin conditions such as eczema and boils.

MAIN USES:

Its oil is useful in treating skin disorders; the seeds in treating respiratory ailments, depression, listlessness.

CYMBOPOGON/LEMON GRASS

Cymbopogon citratus (Gramineae)

HISTORY and USES:

Native from Sri Lanka and South India, lemon grass is now widely cultivated in the tropical areas of America and Asia. Its oil is used as a culinary flavoring primarily in pan-Asian dishes, in perfume, and in herbal medicine. Lemon grass is principally taken as a tea to remedy digestive problems, diarrhea, and general stomach aches. It relaxes the muscles of the stomach and digestive organs, and relieves cramping pains and flatulence. Lemon grass tea can also be helpful in cooling a fever. If applied externally as a salve, a poultice, or as diluted essential oil, it can ease pain associated with arthritis, sore muscles, and sore tendons.

MAIN PROPERTIES:

Digestive, antispasmodic, analgesic, febrifuge

DAISY

Bellis perennis

HISTORY and USES:

Though considered a garden weed, daisies have a varieties of medicinal properties. Daisy extract can be used to treat kidney problems, rheumatism, arthritis, bronchitis and diarrhea. It also has astringent properties as well.

MAIN PROPERTIES:

Anti-inflammatory, astringent

DAMIANA

Turnera diffusa syn. T. diffusa var. aphrodisiaca
(Turneraceae)

HISTORY and USES:

Originally native to the Gulf of Mexico, damiana was used as an aphrodisiac and as stimulant to ease sufferers of mild depression. Damiana has a strong aroma, and a pungent, slightly bitter taste. The tea can also act as a nerve tonic, and as a urinary tract antiseptic.

MAIN PROPERTIES:

Nerve tonic, aphrodisiac, antidepressant, urinary antiseptic.

DANDELION

Taraxacum officinale (Compositae)

HISTORY and USES:

Occurring naturally in Asia, Dandelion is now a common plant and is most often referred to as a garden weed. Arabs, Persians, and East Indians have long been familiar with the dandelion's ability to help the liver. The leaves, which can be eaten raw in salads or as a garnish, are a powerful diuretic. Ingestion of the roots can help the kidneys and the liver detoxify the blood more effectively. It has a high potassium content, and may as such be useful for athletes or physical laborers to prevent muscle cramping and spasms. It also acts like a mild laxative, stimulates the appetite, and eases the process of digestion. Dandelion roots and leaves can be eaten, or made into a tea.

MAIN PROPERTIES:

Diuretic, digestive, antibiotic.

DILL

Anethum graveolens syn. Peucedanum graveolens
(Umbelliferae)

HISTORY and USES:

The ancient Egyptians used dill as an active ingredient in
pain-killing teas and poultices, and the Romans used dill as
a stomach remedy. Dill indeed is an excellent herb for
relieving indigestion, gas, and flatulence. Dill's essential oil
can calm intestinal spasms and griping and helps to settle
colic. The seeds, if chewed, can act as a breath freshener.
Dill makes a useful addition to cough, cold and flu
remedies, and is a mild diuretic. Dill encourages lactation,
and when taken regularly by nursing mothers in the form
of a tea, or just by eating the leaves, helps to prevent colic
in their nursing babies.

MAIN PROPERTIES:

Digestive, breath freshener, colic palliative, antibacterial,
antispasmodic, diuretic.

EPHEDRA

Ephedraceae ephedra

HISTORY and USES:

Ephedra plants can grow wild in dry climates, and are primarily found in the Northern Hemisphere. Ephedra leaves have traditionally been used by indigenous people for a variety of medicinal purposes. It is useful for treating asthma, hay fever, and the common cold. It is also chemically related to amphetamine, and can be used to suppress the appetite and stimulate the metabolism. Ephedra recently became popular in the West as a diet drug. Those who have high blood pressure, eating disorders, or heart conditions should be very wary of using this herb.

MAIN PROPERTIES:

Antihistamine, stimulant, appetite suppressant.

EUCALYPTUS, BLUE GUM

Eucalyptus globulus (Myrtaceae)

HISTORY and USES:

Eucalyptus is native from Australia, and though in use by aboriginal Australian peoples for centuries, eucalyptus is an ingredient in modern-day western medications. Eucalyptus is a powerful antiseptic excellent for relieving coughs and colds, sore throats and other infections. It is, in fact, one of the main active ingredients in Vicks. The leaves cool the body and relive fever. Inhaling the vapors of the essential oils heated in water can clear sinus and bronchial congestions. The essential oil has also strong anti-biotic, anti-viral and anti-fungal action and can be used as a tincture or salve. Eucalyptus can also benefit the skin by encouraging local blood flow.

MAIN PROPERTIES:

Antiseptic, expectorant, stimulates local blood flow, anti-fungal, febrifuge

FENNEL

Foeniculum vulgare (Umbelliferae)

HISTORY and USES:

Fennel was originally native to the Mediterranean and was used by the Greeks and Romans for food, spice and medicine. Chewing fennel seeds can relieve flatulence, but settle colic, stimulate the appetite, and aid in digestion. Fennel is also diuretic and anti-inflammatory. It can also act as an expectorant for those suffering from sinus congestion, colds, or coughs. An infusion of the seeds may be gargled for sore throats and will act as mild expectorant. Fennel increases breast-milk production, and can also be used as an eye wash for conjunctivitis. Essential oil from the sweet variety is used for its digestive and relaxing properties.

MAIN PROPERTIES:

Digestive, antispasmodic, anti-inflammatory, expectorant

FEVERFEW

Tanacetum parthenium

HISTORY and USES:

Feverfew is a traditional medicinal herb. The plant grows into a small bush with citrus-scented leaves and is covered by flowers. As such, the plant can be used for ornamentation as well as medicinal value. It spreads rapidly, and they will cover a wide area after a few years, so it can also be useful for providing ground cover in a large garden. Feverfew has been used for reducing fever, for treating headaches, arthritis and digestive problems. The active ingredients in feverfew include parthenolide and tanetin. Feverfew can easily be found in health food or vitamin stores as tea or caplets, but it might take four to six weeks before they become effective, and feverfew is not an effective for acute migraines. Sufferers of cancer, especially leukemia, and those prone to cold sores, should stay away from feverfew and look to a different herb to use as medicine for the above problems.

MAIN PROPERTIES:

Vasoconstrictor, analgesic, febrifuge

FOXGLOVE

Digitalis purpurea

HISTORY and USES:

Digitalis refers to a genus containing about 20 plants. The use of Digitalis purpurea has long been used in folk medicine to treat arrhythmia, and regulate the speed and rhythm of the heart rate. The part of the plant that is useful for therapeutic purposes comes from the leaves of plants that are at least two years old. Great care must be taken when using this plant for medicinal purposes, however, because it can be quite toxic. Digitalis toxicity results from an overdose of digitalis and causes anorexia, nausea, vomiting and diarrhea, and blurred vision. It was, if you may recall, the poison used against James Bond in the 2006 film Casino Royale. Because a frequent side effect of digitalis is reduction of appetite, some individuals have used the plant as a weight loss aid, but this can be very dangerous due to the potential for abuse or overdose.

The entire plant, if taken incorrectly or in wrong doses, is a poison; including the seeds and roots. Just a swallow can be enough to cause death. Early symptoms of overdose include nausea, vomiting, anorexia, diarrhea, abdominal pain, hallucinations, delirium, and severe headache.

Children have died from drinking from a vase containing digitalis flowers. The plant is also toxic to animals, so it should only be cultivated in a home or garden if great care is taken to keep it away from pets and children.

MAIN PROPERTIES:

Anti-convulsant

GARLIC

Allium sativum (Liliaceae)

HISTORY and USES:

Garlic is originally from central Asia but was used as flavoring and medication by the Egyptians, Greeks, and Romans. Garlic is still incredibly useful. It is one of the most effective anti-biotic plants commonly available, acting on bacteria, viruses and alimentary parasites. The cloves can counter nose, throat and chest, and can act as an expectorant. It will also act as a palliative for congested sinuses and can help clear blocked nasal passages to bring relief in cases of bad allergies or a cold. Garlic is also known to reduce cholesterol, increase circulation, lower blood pressure, and lower blood sugar levels. It can also help to expunge parasites, such as worms, from the body.

MAIN PROPERTIES:

Antibiotic, expectorant, diaphoretic, hypotensive, antispasmodic, vermifuge

GENTIAN

Gentiana lutea (Gentianaceae)

HISTORY and USES:

Native to Europe and Asia Minor, is a powerful, bitter herb that stimulates appetite, increases the production of saliva, increases the production of bile and gastric juices, and thus promotes digestion. It also acts as a gastric anti-inflammatory and kills parasitic worms. Gentian is also used to treat liver and spleen problems and to promote menstruation. It can also ease discomfort or pain associated with poor digestion, inflammation, or irritation of the stomach.

MAIN PROPERTIES:

Bitter, carminative, analgesic, vermifuge

GINGER

Zingiber officinali (Zingiberaceae)

HISTORY and USES:

Ginger is native to Southeast Asia and but is now cultivated elsewhere. Ginger is an important part of some kinds of Asian cuisine and medicine. Ginger can be used to treat a cold and encourage sweating. It brings relief to digestion, stimulates circulation, reduce headaches and kill intestinal parasites. It can also act as a breath freshener, a cough suppressant, and a stimulant.

MAIN PROPERTIES:

Diaphoretic, carminative, circulatory stimulant, cough suppressant, anti-inflammatory, antiseptic.

GINKGO

Ginkgo biloba (Ginkgoaceae)

HISTORY and USES:

Ginkgo is one of the oldest trees on the planet. Though its medicinal properties have long been valued in China, its therapeutic actions have only recently been researched by Western scientist. Gingko has anti microbial and anti inflammatory properties, and has a profound effect on brain function and cerebral circulation. It can prevent dizziness, tinnitus, short-term memory loss, depression and other symptoms of poor circulation of blood in the brain. Its effect on poor circulation also used to treat other related disorders like diabetes, hemorrhoids and varicose veins. Ginkgo is also valuable for asthma, for treating allergies, and as a stimulant. It is sold in health food stores in capsules, and can be taken as supplements. It can also be made into a tea.

MAIN PROPERTIES:

Circulatory stimulant and tonic, anti-asthmatic, antispasmodic, anti-allergenic, anti-inflammatory.

GINSENG

Panax ginseng (Araliaceae)

HISTORY and USES:

Ginseng is native to north-eastern China, eastern Russia and Korea, and has been valued in Eastern medicine for thousands of years. An Arabian physician brought ginseng back to Europe in the 9th century. It has only been fairly recently, however, that westerners realized that it has a tremendous ability to improve stamina and cope with stress. Ginseng increases mental and physical efficiency and resistance to stress and disease. It can act to speed the metabolism, and as such, is a frequent additive to diet pills and appetite suppressants. It can also act as a powerful stimulant, and it is rumored to be an effective aphrodisiac.

MAIN PROPERTIES:

Tonic, stimulant, physical and mental revitalizer.

GOLDENSEAL

Hydrastis Canadensis

HISTORY and USES:

Goldenseal is an herb in the buttercup family. It is a flowering plant that bears a single berry in the summer.

Goldenseal can be effective with used topically as an antimicrobial agent, it can be taken internally as a digestion aid, and it can be made into a mouth wash to treat canker sores. Goldenseal may be purchased in salve, tablet, tincture form, or as a bulk powder. Goldenseal can also be used to amplify the medicinal effects of other herbs.

Native Americans have long used Goldenseal as a wash for ailments of the eye, to treat cancer, and to treat swollen or inflamed breasts. It can be useful to treat gastritis, atonic dyspepsia, constipation, hepatic congestion, cirrhosis, fevers, post partum hemorrhage, goiters, and gallstones

It can also act to stimulate the appetite and fight damage caused to the liver by alcohol abuse or disease. It has an astringent effect on mucous membranes of the upper respiratory tract, the gastrointestinal tract, the bladder, and the skin. Generally a two week maximum dosage is suggested. Taking goldenseal over a long period of time can reduce absorption of B vitamins. It is important to note that goldenseal should be avoided during pregnancy and lactation, and should be avoided by those who suffer chronic inflammation of the intestines. Some also say that goldenseal should only be used if there are no other substitutes available.

MAIN PROPERTIES

Bitter, hepatic, alterative, anti-catarrhal, anti-inflammatory, antimicrobial, laxative

GREEN TEA

Camellia Sinensis

HISTORY AND USES

The beverage green tea is a "true" tea that has been subject to minimal oxidation during processing.

Generally, the tea is brewed with 2.25 grams of tea per 6 ounces of water, or about one teaspoon of green tea per cup. Green tea has been used for thousands of years in Asia to stop bleeding and to help heal wounds, regulate blood sugar, promoting digestion.

Claims that green tea could prevent cancer, treat MS, and boost the metabolism were at first treated by the FDA with skepticism. Eventually, however, after clinical trials, the FDA concluded that an ingredient in green tea would be useful for treating genital warts.

Clinical trials have also proved that green tea can help cardiac function and prevent heart attacks, stroke, and lower the risk of death in general. It was also concluded that the tea had high levels of antioxidants which could possibly prevent or treat cancer, and definitely lower the buildup of plaque in arteries.

MAIN PROPERTIES

Stimulant, anti-oxidant, vulnerary, lowers cholesterol, balances blood sugar, mild appetite suppressant.

GUMPLANT

Grindelia camporum syn. *G. robusta* var. *rigida*
(Compositae)

HISTORY and USES:

Gumplant is native to the south-western US and parts of
Mexico, has been used for centuries by Native Americans
to treat bronchial irritations and rashes stemming from
contact with poison oak. The medicinal value of the plant
was not recognized by western doctors until the mid-l9th
century. Gumplant is an anti-spasmodic and expectorant,
and can lower blood pressure. As such, it is useful in
treating heart conditions, asthma, bronchitis, whooping
cough, hay fever and cystitis. If applied externally as a
poultice or salve, it can relieve and heal skin irritations,
rashes, and burns.

MAIN PROPERTIES:

Anti-spasmodic, expectorant, hypotensive, soothes rashes

HAMAMELIS, WITCH HAZEL

Hamamamelis virginiana (Hamamelidaceae)

HISTORY and USES:

Witch hazel is native to eastern North America, ranging from New England to western Minnesota. It was a traditional remedy of many native North American peoples, and is an active ingredient in cosmetics and salves today. Witch hazel acts mostly on the veins and circulation. As such, it is useful for alleviating pain of bruises, and sore muscles. It can stop bleeding, relieve hemorrhoids, bring down inflammation and swelling in varicose veins, act as a palliative on phlebitis, and relieve the itch and redness of insect bites. American Indians used poultices soaked in a decoction of witch hazel bark to treat tumors and inflammations, especially of the eye, and took the herb internally to alleviate and stem the flow of hemorrhaging and heavy menstrual bleeding. Hammamelis was introduced in Europe on the18th century.

MAIN PROPERTIES:

Astringent, anti-inflammatory, stops external and internal bleeding.

HAWTHORN

Crataegus oxyacantha & *C. monogyna* (Rosaceae)

HISTORY and USES:

Hawthorn is native of Europe with but close relatives of the species have also been found growing wild in parts of Asia and North America. The tree has been known and appreciated by the ancient Greeks, Arabs, and Europeans. Hawthorn is an extremely valuable medicinal herb. The whole plant must be used to guarantee the best level of effectiveness. It can be used to dilate the blood vessels, which is particularly useful when someone is suffering a heart attack or experiencing loss of cardiac function. It can also alleviate feelings of congestions and oppression in the chest region. It serves to increase blood flow to the heart muscles and regulate the heart beat. Recent research done by Western scientists have confirmed that the plant does indeed have such properties, and that relief of these symptoms isn't merely a placebo effect.

MAIN PROPERTIES:

Cardio tonic, diuretic, astringent, relaxant, antioxidant.

HONEY

HISTORY and USES:

For at least 2700 years, honey has been used to treat a
variety of ailments through topical application.
Antibacterial properties of honey are the result of a
hydrogen peroxide like behavior on a chemical level, and
high acidity. Topical honey has been used successfully in a
comprehensive treatment of diabetic ulcers and
antioxidants in honey have been shown to reduce the
damage done to the colon in colitis. Furthermore, some
studies suggest that honey may be effective in increasing
the populations of good bacteria in the digestive tract,
which may help strengthen the immune system, improve
digestion, lower cholesterol, and prevent cancer of the
colon.

Some studies suggest that the topical use of honey may
reduce odors, swelling, and scarring when used to treat
wounds; it may also prevent the dressing from sticking to a
wound that is healing.

MAIN PROPERTIES:

Antiseptic, antibiotic, vulnerary

HORSERADISH

Armoracia rusticana

HISTORY and USES:

The horseradish is a flowering plant that is a relative of the mustard and the cabbage, and has been used in culinary pursuits and medicine since the ancient Egyptians. The horseradish root itself, when dug up from the ground, doesn't have a particularly strong smell. However, once grated or cut, it has a pungent aroma, and must be added to vinegar or it will blacken and become bitter. The roots are a diuretic and urinary tract infections, bronchitis, sinus congestion, and coughs.

MAIN PROPERTIES:

Diuretic, expectorant

HYSSOP

Hyssopus officinalis (Labiatae)

HISTORY and USES:

Hyssop is native to the Mediterranean region and currently is commercially cultivated in Europe, Russia and India. Hyssop is potentially useful as both a soothing agent and a tonic, and can act as an anti-spasmodic. It is used to treat cough, bronchitis, respiratory catarrh, asthma, difficulties in breathing, sore throats and the common cold. As a sedative, hyssop is a useful remedy against asthma in both children and adults, especially where the condition accompanied by a lot of mucous congestion. Hyssop is also a valuable culinary herb, and is used to flavor various liqueurs, including Chartreuse.

MAIN PROPERTIES:

Anti-spasmodic, expectorant, diaphoretic, anti-inflammatory, hepatic.

IPECAC SYRUP

Psychotria ipecacuanha

HISTORY and USES:

Ipecac syrup is made from the roots of the ipecacuanha plant. It is native to Brazil, and is used as an emetic in folk medicine. It is also valuable as a diaphoretic, nauseate, and expectorant as well. It is an almost indispensable item to have in a medicine cabinet if there are small children in the house. Should a child (or adult) ingest poison, call poison control immediately. They will generally instruct you on how to administer ipecac to induce vomiting in the child (or adult).

MAIN PROPERTIES:

Emetic, expectorant

JASMINE

Jasminum grandiflorum (Oleaceae)

HISTORY and USES:

Jasmine is most likely originally native to Iran or the North Eastern Arabian peninsula, and is now well known and cultivated in most of the world. It is still used extensively in perfumery and cosmetics. Syrup made from the flowers can be very useful for calming coughs, and tea made from the leaves can be used to rinse sore eyes and clean out wounds. Jasmine flowers make a calming infusion that has a sedative effect, and can be taken to relieve tension. The oil is considered antidepressant and relaxant. It is used externally to soothe dry and sensitive skin.

MAIN PROPERTIES:

Aromatic, anti-spasmodic, expectorant, vulnerary

JUNIPER

Juniperus communis (Cupressaceae)

HISTORY and USES:

Juniper is found in Europe, south-western Asia, and parts of North America. Juniper is a tonic, a diuretic and can be antiseptic within the urinary tract. It is a very useful remedy for cystitis, and can act as a diuretic to relieve fluid retention, but should be avoided in cases of kidney disease or weak kidneys. In the digestive system, juniper can ease colic, support the function of the stomach, and settle indigestion. Taken internally or applied externally, juniper is helpful in the treatment of chronic arthritis, gout, and rheumatic conditions. Applied externally as a diluted essential oil, it has a slightly warming effect on the skin, increasing circulation and possibly aiding in the expulsion of toxins and wastes.

MAIN PROPERTIES:

Diuretic, anti-microbial, carminative, anti-rheumatic.

KOREAN MINT/PURPLE GIANT HYSSOP

Agastache rugosa

HISTORY and USES:

Korean mint has long been a vital herb in Chinese medicine. The flowers and leaves of the plant can be made into a decoction to treat problems with digestion. It promotes sweating, and also can prevent nausea or vomiting, and can prevent or alleviate diarrhea. It can also be made into a tea to treat or prevent fever, and has anti-fungal and antibacterial properties. It can soothe hyperactivity and restlessness, as well as insomnia, because it acts as a mild sedative.

MAIN PROPERTIES:

Antiemetic, antidiarrhea, antipyretic, diaphoretic, anti-fungal, antibacterial, mild sedative, anti-spasmodic

LAUREL, BAY LAUREL

Laurus nobilis (Lauraceae)

HISTORY and USES:

Laurel is originally native to the Mediterranean region but is now cultivated all over the world. In ancient Greek and Rome, bay laurel was sacred to the gods Apollo and Aesculapius, who together supervised and acted as patrons of healing and medicine. The herb was thought to be greatly protective and healing. An infusion of the leaves can be taken for its warming and tonic effect on the stomach and bladder, and a plaster made from the leaves was used to relieve the swelling and pain associated with wasp and bee stings. Bay laurel is also useful in treating upper digestive tract disorders and to ease arthritic aches, pains, and swelling. It is settling to the stomach and has a tonic effect, stimulating the appetite and the secretion of digestive juices.

MAIN PROPERTIES:

Astringent, digestive, insect stings

LAVENDER

Lavandula officinalis syn. *L. angustifolia* (Labiatae)

HISTORY and USES:

Lavender is native to the Mediterranean region but is now widely cultivated. It is, to this day, used in cosmetics, perfumery, and in cooking. Lavender tea can help cure headaches, especially when caused by stress. It can also uplift the mood and help to palliate the symptoms of depression. Externally, lavender oil can be used as a stimulating liniment to help ease aches and pains of rheumatism. It can also dilate the blood vessels, stimulate circulation, and relieve muscle spasms.

MAIN PROPERTIES:

Carminative, relieves muscle spasms, antidepressant, antiseptic and antibacterial, stimulates blood flow.

LEMON

Citrus Limon (Rutaceae)

HISTORY and USES:

A native from Asia, it was first introduced to Europe by the Arabs when they were in control of Spain. It is now widely cultivated in Italy, California and Australia. It is an important and versatile natural medicine. It is cheap, readily available, and can easily be used at home. Lemons have a high vitamin C content that helps improve resistance to infection, and can reduce the duration of a cold or flu. It is taken as a preventative for stomach infections, circulatory problems and arteriosclerosis. Lemon juice and oil are effective in killing germs. Lemon juice also decreases inflammation and improves digestion. Drinking a cup of lemon tea can help soothe a fever and eating a lemon slice can help relieve sinus congestion.

MAIN PROPERTIES:

Antiseptic, anti-rheumatic, antibacterial, antioxidant reduces fever.

LICORICE/LIQUORICE

Glycyrrhiza glabra

HISTORY and USES:

Liquorice has been cultivated in Europe and China for medicinal purposes for centuries. The roots and leaves can both be used in medicine, as can liquorice extract.

Liquorice extract is produced by boiling liquorice root and evaporating most of the water. Its active principle is glycyrrhizin, a natural sweetener more than 50 times as sweet as sucrose (table sugar).

Powdered liquorice root can be used with good results as an expectorant, and modern cough syrups often include liquorice extract as an active ingredient. It also can be used as a mouthwash or tea to treat cold sores in the mouth. Liquorice is also a mild laxative and may be used as a topical antiviral wash for shingles, and for opthalmic, oral, or genital herpes.

Liquorice can also regulate smooth functioning of the hypothalamus and pituitary glands. It can also be used for immune deficiency disorders, including lupus, scleroderma, and arthritis. Some also report is as effective in combating the symptoms of animal allergies

Liquorice is used in Chinese herbalism as an essential part of anti-cancer formulas.

Eating black liquorice may result in stool that is vivid green in color, which can be entertaining at best and disturbing at worst. Caution should be used when consuming liquorice extract as it can be damaging to the liver.

MAIN PROPERTIES:

Anti inflammatory, expectorant, treatment for cold sores.

MALVA, COMMON MALLOW

Malva silvestris (Malvaceae)

HISTORY and USES:

The young leaves and shoots of this plant have been used in medicine and cooking for hundreds of years. The flowers and leaves are an emollient and can benefit dry or sensitive skin. It is applied as a poultice to reduce swelling and draw out toxins in the event of an insect or spider bite. Taken internally, the leaves reduce stomach and intestinal irritation and have a laxative effect. When common mallow is combined with eucalyptus, it can serve as a remedy for coughs, colds, congestion, and other chest ailments.

MAIN PROPERTIES:

Anti-inflammatory, emollient, astringent, laxative.

MARJORAM, WILD MARJORAM

Origanum vulgare (Labiatae)

HISTORY and USES:

Native from Asia, marjoram is now cultivated
commercially in many regions of the glob. Marjoram tea is
an age-old remedy to aid in digestion, encourage sweating,
and bring on menstruation. If marjoram is placed in hot
water and the steam inhaled, the fumes will clears the
sinuses, break up chest congestion, and relieve laryngitis.
Wild marjoram can help in settling flatulence and can
stimulate the flow of bile. Strongly antiseptic, it may be
taken to treat coughs, tonsillitis, bronchitis and asthma.
The diluted oil can be applied to take away the pain of a
toothache or to soothe painful joints.

MAIN PROPERTIES:

Antiseptic, anti-spasmodic, digestive.

MATE

*Hex paraguariensi*s syn. *I. paraguensis* (Aquifoliaceae)

HISTORY and USES:

Native to South America mate is a traditional South American tea. It has a pleasant aroma, and can act as a substitute to coffee as it increases short-term physical and mental energy levels. It stimulates the nervous system, is mildly analgesic and can have a diuretic effect. Mate can be used to treat headaches, migraines, neuralgic and rheumatic pain, fatigue, listlessness, and mild depression. It has also been used in the treatment of diabetes.

MAIN PROPERTIES:

Stimulant, diuretic, analgesic.

MELISSA, LEMON BALM

Melissa officinalis (Labiatae)

HISTORY and USES:

Lemon Balm has been cultivated in the Mediterranean region for more than 2,000 years. The Muslim herbalist and philosopher Avicenna used lemon balm to treat heart problems. It can also act to calm nervous spasms, colics and heart spasms. Making a tea of it can promote sweat that that is good to treat colds, flus, sinus infections, and fevers. Its sedative action can also assist sufferers of mania and psychosis. Lemon's balm anti-histamine properties is also useful to treat eczema, allergies, and headaches. Today, this sweet-smelling herb is still widely valued for its calming properties and perfumery, and research shows that it can be useful in treating cold sores.

MAIN PROPERTIES:

Relaxant, antispasmodic, increases sweating, carminative, anti-viral, nerve tonic.

MISTLETOE

Viscum album (Loranthaceae)

HISTORY and USES:

Native to Europe and northern Asian, mistletoe can be used to lower blood pressure and heart rate, ease the symptoms of anxiety, and help sufferers of insomnia or other sleep problems. It can also be helpful in cases of panic attacks, headaches, and improves the ability to concentrate. Mistletoe is also prescribed for tinnitus and epilepsy. It may be used to treat hyperactivity in children. Mistletoe contains viscotoxins that inhibit tumors and stimulate the immune system. For this reason, research has been carried out on its potential use as a cancer treating plant.

MAIN PROPERTIES:

Tranquilizer, reduces pain, controls blood pressure.

MOTHERWORT

Leonurus cardiaca (Labiatae)

HISTORY and USES:

Motherwort is native to Europe, and was used as a medicinal plant in early Greece, where it was used to calm sufferers of anxiety. It can also be used to regulate a heart beat, or to encourage cardiac function. Other uses include the improvement of fertility, the relief of postpartum depression, and relief from the symptoms of menopause. It can lower blood pressure, and is an anti-spasmodic and a sedative, and promotes relaxation without drowsiness. Motherwort should not be taken by pregnant women as it stimulates the muscles of the uterus, and is particularly suitable for delayed periods, period pain and premenstrual tension.

MAIN PROPERTIES:

Nerve tonic, anti-spasmodic, hepatic, hypotensive, cardiac tonic.

MUGWORT

Artemesia vulgaris

HISTORY and USES:

Mugwort is related to wormwood, and has some of the same characteristics. The leaves and buds can be used as a seasoning, and in Middle Europe, is used primarily to season goose. In the Middle Ages, it was used to season beer. Mugwort is also used in Korea and Japan to color pancakes and rice cakes.

The plant contains flavonoids, triterpenes, and coumarin derivatives. Chewing some leaves will have an invigorating effect, and will stimulate the nervous system. It should be avoided by pregnant women because it stimulates uterine contractions, and in fact, was used in folk medicine to cause abortion.

MAIN PROPERTIES:

Stimulant, abortifacient

MYRRH

Commiphora molmol syn. *C. myrrha* (Burseraceae)

HISTORY and USES:

Native to the north eastern regions of Africa, myrrh is still found in Ethiopia, Somalia, the Arabian Peninsula, Iran and Thailand. Myrrh has been used for centuries in perfumery, incense and embalming. It can act as an astringent, and has antimicrobial and antiseptic properties which can treat acne and boils as well as mild inflammation and swelling. It is specifically useful in the treatment of infections or sores in the mouth such as ulcers, and gingivitis. It can be used as well to treat catarrhal problems associated with laryngitis and sinusitis.

MAIN PROPERTIES:

Stimulant, antiseptic, anti-inflammatory, astringent, expectorant, antispasmodic, carminative.

NETTLE

Urtica

HISTORY and USES:

The word "nettle" describes about thirty plants within the genus Urtica. Some of them have poisonous tips which can cause severe skin irritations or even death to small animals and livestock. Nettle has long been used as a galactagogue, and can also act as a diuretic. Extracts can be used to treat arthritis, anemia, hay fever, kidney problems, and pain. Nettle is used in hair shampoos to control dandruff, and is said to make hair healthier and shinier. It can also be used to treat an enlarged prostate gland.

MAIN PROPERTIES:

Galactagogue, diuretic, anti-inflammatory

NUTMEG

Myristica fragrans/argentea/otoba

HISTORY and USES:

The essential oil taken from steaming ground nutmeg is currently used often in cosmetics and perfumery. There is anecdotal evidence that nutmeg and nutmeg oil can treat problems of the nervous and digestive systems.

Externally, the oil can be topically applied to provide relief from rheumatic pain and can be applied to an infected or decayed tooth to quell the pain. Using a few drops of nutmeg oil on a sugar lump, a small piece of fruit, or in a teaspoon of honey or maple syrup can act as a cure for nausea, gastroenteritis, chronic diarrhea, and indigestion.

A massage oil to treat muscle pain and ache can be made by mixing 10 drops of nutmeg in 10 ml almond oil.

No more than a few drops of nutmeg oil should be taken internally at a time. In doses exceeding more than a few teaspoons, extreme pain, dehydration, or even death can result. Even three teaspoons can act as a psychedelic drug. Don't get too excited, however, because constipation and inability to urinate, as well as a variety of other unpleasant side effects, can occur if it is used for this purpose.

Nutmeg is an abortifacient, and as such any significant doses should be avoided by pregnant women, or women trying to become pregnant.

MAIN PROPERTIES

Abortifacient, emollient, anti-inflammatory, pain killer.

OATMEAL

HISTORY and USES:

"oatmeal" is used to describe any crushed or rolled oats from a variety of species of plants. It is an excellent, gentle food to eat when convalescing or ill. It can also be made into a paste to ease itching, hives, or insect bites. Dissolving it in the bath will soothe sunburned skin.

MAIN PROPERTIES:

Anti-inflammatory

ONION

Allium cepa

HISTORY and USES:

This popular household food is native to Central Asia, and evidence suggests that onions may be effective in treating the common cold, heart disease, and diabetes. They can act as anti-inflammatory, and have anti-cholesterol, anticancer, and antioxidant components. In homeopathy, onion is used for rhino rhea and hay fever.

Onions are very rich in chromium, a mineral that helps cells respond to insulin, plus vitamin C, and numerous flavonoids.

The higher the intake of onion, the lower the level of glucose found during oral or intravenous glucose tolerance tests. This means that onions could possibly be helpful in controlling spikes in blood sugar.

The regular consumption of onions has, like garlic, been shown to lower high cholesterol levels and high blood pressure, and to be a very effective anti-inflammatory and expectorant. In addition, quercitin and other flavonoids found in onions work with vitamin C to help kill harmful bacteria.

MAIN PROPERTIES

Antiseptic, anti-inflammatory, expectorant

OREGANO

Oreganum vulgare

HISTORY and USES:

Oregano is high in antioxidant activity, and has demonstrated antimicrobial activity against food-borne pathogens. In the Philippines, oregano is not commonly used for cooking but is rather considered as a primarily medicinal plant, useful for relieving children's coughs.

MAIN PROPERTIES:

Expectorant, antioxidant, antiseptic

PASSION FLOWER

Passiflora

HISTORY and USES:

Passion flower is a genus of about 500 species of plants. The leaves and roots of these plants have a long history of use among Native Americans. The fresh or dried leaves are used to make a tea that is used to treat insomnia, hysteria, depression, anxiety and epilepsy, and is also an effective analgesic. The leaves and the roots of some of these types of plants have been used to enhance the effects of psychedelic drugs.

MAIN PROPERTIES

Anti convulsant, analgesic

QUININE

HISTORY and USES:

Quinine today can be manufactured synthetically, but it was first extracted from the bark of the South American cinchona tree. It was used by the local native peoples as a muscle relaxant, and when it was eventually introduced to Europe, was used to treat malaria. Some say that the discovery of quinine as a malaria treatment made it possible for Europeans to settle and colonize Africa. Quinine is currently available in the US with a prescription, and is used to treat arthritis pain. In very large doses, quinine also acts as an abortifacient.

MAIN PROPERTIES:

Analgesic, anti-inflammatory

RASPBERRY

Rubus idaeus

HISTORY and USES:

Raspberries contain measurable and significant amounts of chemicals linked to promoting endothelial and cardiovascular health. Raspberries are considered a high-fiber food, an excellent source of vitamin C and manganese, a good source of vitamin K, and a good source of magnesium. Raspberries are also rich in iron, potassium, and calcium. Raspberries also rank near the top of all fruits for antioxidant strength and concentration.

Though no full-scale academic studies have been undertaken in order to verify the medicinal effectiveness of raspberries for treating a variety of conditions, there are preliminary studies that suggest good results. Raspberries and raspberry leaves can be used to treat microbe infections, inflammation, acute pain, cancer, cardiovascular disease, diabetes, allergies, mild dementia and general decline in cognitive abilities, and degeneration of eyesight with aging.

A cup of raspberry tea daily is recommended by Jethro Kloss, author of the wonderful, thorough herbal medicine book Our Time in Eden. He claims that it will promote general health and well being, and in my experience, this is so.

MAIN PROPERTIES:

Antioxidant, microbial killer, anti inflammatory, blood sugar balancer, vitamin and mineral source.

RED CLOVER

Trifolium pratense

HISTORY and USES:

Red clover is a species of clover that is native to parts of Europe, Asia, and Africa. Red Clover has been used to treat the symptoms of menopause but women who are pregnant and breastfeeding should avoid Red Clover. Red can be used for therapeutic purposes for coughs, bronchitis, eczema, sores, scrofula and can be gargled for mouth ulcers and sore throats. Native Americans have used it in conjunction with goldenseal as a treatment for cancer.

MAIN PROPERTIES:

Expectorant, anti-cancer, sooths ulcers

ROSEMARY

Rosmarinus officinalis

HISTORY and USES:

Rosemary is a member of the mint family, and is native to the Mediterranean. Rosemary, in the dried form, is extremely high in iron, calcium, and Vitamin B6. Rosemary tea can help gout if used as a topical wash or rub. The oil can also be a powerful convulsant.

MAIN PROPERTIES:

Convulsant

SAW PALMETTO

Serenoa Repens

HISTORY and USES:

Saw palmetto, also referred to as serenoa plant, is a small palm, normally reaching a height of around four to seven feet. It is extremely slow growing, and long lived, and some currently growing plants are easily over 700 years old.

Saw palmetto is a fan palm. Saw palmetto extract, taken from the red fruit that the palmetto plant bears, is effective in managing enlarged prostate glands. It can also treat problems with the urinary tract. For some, it is also a very effective aphrodisiac. Those with high cholesterol, however, should consult with a doctor before taking saw palmetto extract.

MAIN PROPERTIES

Anti inflammatory, aphrodisiac.

SKULLCAP

Scutellaria lateriflora

HISTORY and USES:

Plants from the genus Scutellaria are very useful. There are 200 different species of Skullcap and they are not all used in the same way.

Blue Skullcap and Common Skullcap can act as a mild sedative, and can be taken in the form of herbal teas, tablets, or capsules. The oil from the flowers can be used as a nerve tonic and anticonvulsant.
Blue Skullcap is also known to prevent the recurrence of seizure.

MAIN PROPERTIES:

Sedative, anti-convulsant

TEA TREE OIL

Melaleuca alternifolia

HISTORY and USES:

Tea tree oil or melaleuca oil is essential oil taken from the leaves of the Melaleuca alternifolia tree. This tree is native to Australia. Tea tree oil should not be confused with oil from the tea plant, as they have very different qualities. Tea tree oil has been recognized as a potent antiseptic in Australian aboriginal folk medicine for centuries. The scientific and medical communities have done research that supports most of the claims made by Aboriginal communities.

Tea tree oil is an antifungal agent, and if a few drops are added to a shampoo, it can also treat dandruff. It also has anti-viral properties, and can kill Candida. It is an excellent astringent, and if diluted and applied to the skin, it can be a very effective treatment for oily skin and acne.

Tea tree oil is also effective for treating insect bites, ringworm, boils and minor wounds. It can also soothe sunburns, ear infections, and bee stings.

Toothpastes, dentifrices, and mouthwashes containing tea tree oil can treat bad breath, gum disease, and canker sores.

Tea tree oil has a very pungent smell and is very powerful. It can act as an irritant, so before applying it topically to a sensitive area of the skin, it should be tested to make sure there will be no severe reaction. If used to treat acne, dandruff, cold sores, fungus, or yeast infections, it should be greatly diluted. Great, great caution should be used in treating ear infections with tea tree oil, as it can be very hard on the eardrum and membrane.

MAIN PROPERTIES:

Anti-fungal, anti-bacterial, anti-viral, disinfectant, mild vulnerary

THYME

Thymus L

HISTORY and USES:

There are about 350 plants that fit into the genus "thymus". It was widely used for embalming in ancient Egypt, and was used by the ancient Greeks to freshen and purify rooms. Currently, it is primarily known as a useful culinary herb, though it does have some medicinal properties.

The essential oil of common thyme is an antiseptic, and is antifungal.

A tea made by infusing the herb in water can be used for to treat coughs, irritations of the respiratory tract, and bronchitis. Because it is antiseptic, thyme boiled in water and cooled can be gargled to soothe a sore throat. Thyme tea can cause uterine contractions, and as such, should not be taken by pregnant women.

MAIN PROPERTIES:

Antiseptic, antifungal, anti-inflammatory, expectorant

VALERIAN

Valeriana officinalis

HISTORY and USES:

Valerian usually refers to a herb or dietary supplement prepared from roots of the plant, which can be sold in teas or capsules.

Valerian has historically been used as a sedative, anti-convulsant, migraine treatment and pain reliever. Valerian is used against sleeping disorders, restlessness and anxiety, and as a muscle relaxant. It is also used traditionally to treat gastrointestinal pain and spastic colitis. One study found that valerian tends to sedate the agitated person and stimulate the fatigued person, bringing about a balancing effect on the system.

MAIN PROPERTIES:

Anticonvulsant, relaxant, sedative, pain reliever.

WHEAT GRASS

HISTORY and USES:

Wheatgrass is a plant of the genus Caroline that can be made into juice or eaten as-is. Wheatgrass, whether in juice or eaten as raw leaves, provides chlorophyll, amino acids, minerals, vitamins, and enzymes. Some claim that regular consumption of wheatgrass can prevent or treat cancer; these claims are not substantiated by medical trials. Wheatgrass does, however, contain a wide variety of beneficial vitamins and minerals

MAIN PROPERTIES:

Good source of fiber, nutrition

WHITE VINEGAR

HISTORY and USES:

Vinegar can be used as a herbicide if diluted to 20%
vinegar and 80% water. It may kill some top growth if a
plant is particularly delicate, but will not kill the roots.
Vinegar along with hydrogen peroxide is used in the
livestock industry to kill bacteria and viruses before
refrigeration storage. Hippocrates prescribed vinegar for
many ailments, from skin rash to ear infection. Multiple
trials indicate that taking vinegar with food increases
satiety dramatically, and even a single application of
vinegar can lead to reduced food intake for a whole day.
Small amounts of vinegar—i.e. two tablespoons per
serving--added to food, or taken along with a meal, have
been shown by to reduce the glycemic index of
carbohydrate food for people with and without diabetes.

MAIN PROPERTIES

Antiseptic, pesticide, appetite suppressant, fungicide.

WHITE WILLOW BARK

Salix alba

HISTORY and USES:

Hippocrates wrote extensively about a bitter powder extracted from willow bark that could ease aches and pains and reduce fevers. White willow bark, often an ingredient in many pharmaceuticals today, can be used very effectively in place of aspirin or Tylenol. Native American Indians used it for headaches, fever, sore muscles, rheumatism, and chills. Salicin—contained in the bark of a white willow tree-- like aspirin, is a chemical derivative of salicylic acid.

MAIN PROPERTIES:

Vaso constrictor, pain killer, fever reducer

YARROW

Achillea millefolium

HISTORY and USES:

Achillea millefolium or Yarrow is a flowering plant found native to many parts of the Northern Hemisphere. Yarrow decoctions have been used to treat inflammations such as hemorrhoids, and headaches. Infusions of Yarrow, used either internally or externally, can hasten recovery from severe bruising. The most medicinally active part of the plant are the flowering tops, and today, yarrow is used primarily to treat colds and influenza, and problems with the circulatory and digestive tracts.

The flowers can be dried and made into a tea for a very effective treatment of severe allergies, and as an expectorant for respiratory phlegm. The same tea can be used as a wash for eczema. The essential oil of yarrow can be used as an anti-inflammatory, a massage oil for inflamed joints, or in chest rubs for colds and influenza.

The leaves can also act as a diuretic, a fever reducer, and to stimulate menstruation. Yarrow can be used with many other herbs and will magnify their healing properties. This extremely versatile herb can be used to treat amenorrhea, joint inflammation, tissue inflammation, colds, chicken pox, circulation, digestive disorders, dyspepsia, eczema, fevers, gastritis, and, influenza. It can cat as an insect repellant, as a stimulant, and as a clotting agent to stem the flow of internal bleeding. Some say that it can induce a miscarriage or act as birth control, but studies have yet to prove this. As such, pregnant or lactating women should stay away from it, but women seeking a natural birth control method may want to study up on other herbs that have been through clinical trials.

Yarrow can be an excellent garden plant because it repels insects and attracts wasps, bees, and ladybugs.

MAIN PROPERTIES:

Blood clotter, stimulant, pain killer, menstruation inducer, fever reducer.

YOGHURT CULTURES

L. acidophilus, Lactobacillus casei, Bifidobacterium

HISTORY and USES:

Yoghurt or yogurt is a dairy product produced by bacterial fermentation of milk. There is evidence that yogurt has been produced in Eastern Europe for over 4000 years. For centuries, yogurt was used by the Turkish to treat a variety of ailments, including diarrhea.

Yoghurt is made by introducing specific bacteria strains into milk that is then fermented. In order for a milk product to be considered "yogurt" by the FDA, it must include specific kinds of bacteria, including L. acidophilus, Lactobacillus casei and Bifidobacterium species.

L. acidophilus naturally inhabits the intestines and vagina and protect against some unhealthy organisms and "bad" bacteria L. acidophilus also tends to consume the nutrients many other harmful microorganisms eat, therefore reducing their ability to live in the digestive tract. During digestion, L. acidophilus also assists in the production of niacin, folic acid, and pyridoxine. These bacteria can boost the immune system, and can be consumed through yogurt to treat yeast infections. Some people report L. acidophilus provides relief from indigestion and diarrhea

Yogurt is a very effective way to treat a yeast infection because L. acidophilus is part of the normal vaginal flora. The acid produced by L. acidophilus in the vagina helps to control the growth of the fungus Candida albicans, which causes yeast infections. Often, after taking large doses of antibiotics or consuming large quantities of sugar, women will suffer from yeast infections.

For those who do not like the taste of yogurt, L. acidophilus is often sold in health stores in pill or powder form.

Lactobacillus casei is beneficial because it encourages the growth of desirable bacteria. This particular species of lactobacillus is documented to have It is known to improve digestion and reduce intolerance to lactose.

MAIN PROPERTIES:

Anti-fungal

GLOSSARY OF TERMS

This book attempts to introduce the beginning herbalist to the possibilities of herbal medicine and folk remedies. Words like "tea" and "brew" may be familiar, but words like "decoction" or "tincture" may not. Therefore, I have included a glossary of terms that will help you understand this book better.

ANALGESIC: medicine given to ease pain

ANTICONVULSANT: An agent that can prevent or arrest seizures and tremors.

ANTIFUNGAL: A substance that kills fungus, usually applied topically.

ANTIOXIDANT: a substance that prevents cellular damage caused by free radicals.

ANTISEPTIC: A substance that prevents, retards, or destroys microorganisms.

ANTISPASMODIC: an agent that calms or reduces muscle spasms or cramps.

ASTRINGENT: An agent high in tannins that can shrink tissue. This is especially useful for controlling or stopping bleeding.

CARMINATIVE: An agent that relieves and removes gas from the digestive system, and aids in digestion.

DECOCTION: A liquid, much like a tea, made from boiling part of a plant in water. Usually, the type of plant or part of the plant will be bark, roots, stems, or other woody parts. A decoction is similar to an infusion, but stronger because the plant will usually stay in the water longer than 10 – 20 minutes.

DIAPHORETIC: an agent that encourages sweating

EMOLLIENT: substance that softens or smoothes the skin

EMMENOGOGUE: substance that causes or encourages menstruation.

EXPECTORANT: A substance that makes mucous easier to cough up from the lungs or upper respiratory tract.

FEBRIFUGE: an agent that reduces fever.

FLAVONOID: a group of chemicals with antioxidant properties found only in vascular plants.

HYPOTENSIVE: an agent that lowers blood pressure.

INFUSION: A tea-like liquid made from boiling plant parts in water for 10 to 20 minutes.

SEDATIVE: a substance that reduces or calms nervous tension

TEA: a liquid made from pouring hot water herbs (usually dried) and letting them sit for ten minutes or so. A tea is not as strong as a decoction or infusion.

TONIC: a substance that acts to invigorate or strengthen.

VERMIFUGE: a substance that can kill or expel worms.

VULNERARY: a substance that hastens the regeneration of tissue, helping to heal wounds quickly.

PARTICULARLY USEFUL HERBS

It is not always practical, nor fiscally possible to keep every single medicinal herb in the home at all times. I recommend, however, always having the following on hand:

Tea tree oil

Cinnamon

Ginger

Lemon

Spearmint/peppermint

Cayenne pepper

HERBS TO BE AVOIDED BY PREGNANT WOMEN

Of course, it is expected that a pregnant woman would check with her doctor before medicating herself, even if the medication is herbal. But this section has been included as a just-in-case. Also, as an interesting historical aside, women have long used herbs and spices as birth control. Some herbs prevent implantation of the fertilized egg. Others cause abortion. It is rumored that Middle Eastern women would use apricot kernels as IUDs, but this is merely folklore.

In any case, herbs listed as emmenagogues are substances which have the ability to provoke menstruation. As such, they should never be taken by pregnant women. But a woman who is late on her period for other reasons could benefit from the use of these herbs. It should be noted that an emmenagogue is not necessarily an abortifacient. An emmenagogue is an herb which encourages menstrual bleeding, and abortifacient herbs do this as well, but are stronger, and may stimulate uterine contractions.

Mild Emmenagogues:

Parsley, Ginger, Yarrow, Feverfew, Rosemary and Sage.

Medium Strength Emmenagogues:

Parsley, Queen Anne's Lace Seeds, Black Cohosh, Mugwort, Juniper.

Strong Emmenagogues :

Pennyroyal, Angelica, Savin, Rue, Tansy, Asafetida, Blue Cohosh, and Vitamin C, celery seed, birthwort.

Uterine Contracting Herbs:

Blue Cohosh, Cotton Seed/Root, Angelica, Tansy, Mugwort, Juniper berries, Chamomile.

Uterine stimulating herbs:

Angelica, Black Cohosh, Ginger, Horseradish, Queen Anne's Lace Seeds/Root

Potential herbal contraceptives:

Cotton Root, Juniper Root, Queen Anne's Lace Seeds

USEFUL RECIPES

The following section is a list of home remedies that are
especially useful, and fairly easy to make. Most use
ingredients that can be commonly found in most
households, and almost all grocery stores.

ROSEMARY TEA

Useful for: general aches and pains, lack of energy

Directions: boil water, and add one teaspoon of crushed or dried rosemary. Pour through a strainer and serve. Honey may be used as a sweetener

GINGER TEA

Useful for: asthma, respiratory problems

Directions: add ¼ teaspoon of ginger to ½ cup of hot water. Take two tablespoons before bedtime.

HOLY BASIL TEA

Useful for: chronic bronchitis; chronic irritation of the upper respiratory tract

1 tablespoon of basil
2 cups of hot water.

Directions: Take two tablespoons four times per day

CINNAMON TEA

Useful for: congestion; common cold

3 g. bark
1 ½ cups of hot water.

Directions: Steep and drink at bedtime as tea.

CAYENNE PEPPER SHOT

Useful for: extreme congestion, sinus infection

1 c. hot water.

1 tsp lemon juice

1 garlic clove put through a garlic press

1 pinch cayenne pepper.

Directions: Mix well and take as a shot.

FENNEL LINSEED TEA

Useful for: constipation

1/3 teaspoon Fennel seeds, powdered
1/3 teaspoon Linseed seeds, powdered
1/3 teaspoon Liquorice root, powdered
1 3/4 cups Water

Directions: Combine equal quantities of the three herbs and add this herb mixture to the water and boil, covered, for 10 minutes. Filter the tea before drinking.

Dosage: 1 cup, 3 times a day.

BLACK PEPPER TEA

Useful for: diarrhea

5 crushed pepper seeds
1 c. water
Directions: Boil the seeds in the water for 15 minutes in a covered container. Remove from the heat and strain. Take 1/2 teaspoon, twice a day.

GINGER MINT TEA

Useful for: fever

2g crushed ginger

2g crushed mint leaves

1 ½ c. hot water

Directions: Mix the 2 herbs in the water and bring to a boil. Cover and cook for 15 minutes. Strain the decoction and drink.

LEMON TEA

Useful for: cold, fever

1 lemon slice

1 cup hot water

Directions: bring water to a boil. Pour a cup and add the lemon slice. Sip slowly.

YARROW TEA

Useful for: piles

1-2 tea spoon Herb/blossoms, crushed
1 cup Water

Directions: prepare the infusion by combining the herb with the water in a covered container. Let the mixture stand for 5-6 hours. Strain before drinking.

CORIANDER INFUSION

Useful for: impotence

1 teaspoon chopped Coriander Leaves
1 cup Boiling water

Directions: To make the infusion, cover the leaves with boiling water, close the lid of the teapot and leave for 15 minutes, then strain.

Dosage: 2-4 table spoon a day.

Remember: coriander leaf extract acts as an aphrodisiac, while, Coriander seed extract suppresses the sex drive.

MINT TEA

Useful for: stomach pain

1 tea spoon spearmint leaves, crushed
2 cups Water

Directions: Combine the spearmint leaves and the water
and raise the mixture to a boil in a covered container.
Remove from the heat and let the tea stand for 15 minutes.
Strain before drinking.

Dosage: 1-2 cups a day.

GINGER INFUSION

Useful for: painful menstruation

6 g Embelia, whole plant, powdered

6 g Ginger, dried, powdered

1 3/4 cups Water

6 g Sugar

Directions: Mix the two herbs and boil. Remove from the heat, strain and sweeten with the sugar.

Dosage: 3/4 cup a day.

ONION COLD RELIEF

Useful for: extreme congestion; chest colds

1 onion, sliced

Merely keep the sliced onion by the bed of a person who is suffering from horrific chest congestion. A personal testimonial: I once was so sick that I couldn't sleep unless I was sitting up. Otherwise I would be overcome with wracking coughs. I tried everything: codeine, robitussin, liquor, lemon juice, a cayenne pepper shot, a chest rub...nothing worked. I could not sleep. Finally I received a suggestion to slice an onion and leave it by my bed. My room smelled for three days, but I was finally able to sleep peacefully.

NATURAL FLU RELIEF

Useful for: relief from the flu

2 teaspoons cayenne pepper

1 ½ teaspoons salt

1 cup hot chamomile tea

1 cup apple cider vinegar

juice from 1 lemon slice

Directions: Make chamomile tea. While it is steeping, grind the cayenne pepper and salt together. Add the hot chamomile tea, let it cool, and then add the vinegar.

Dosage: Take a tablespoon or so every half hour.

INDEX:

Lightning Source UK Ltd.
Milton Keynes UK
UKOW040046030113

204317UK00001B/20/P